J

D1162770

613.2
Vin

Jefferson Davis Parish Library

DISCARD

Vine, Jonathan,
Clean food diet : + 50 best recipes
118 W Plaquemine St.
Jennings, LA 70546
19.00   Jennings
Amazon   12/08/2015

Clean Food Diet

+ 50 Best Recipes

Clean Food Diet

+ 50 Best Recipes

By

Jonathan Vine

Clean Food Diet\ Jonathan Vine

Editor: Hofit Carmi

ISBN-13: 978-1502911971

ISBN-10: 1502911973

Copyright© 2014 by Jonathan Vine
All rights reserved. No part of this book may be reproduced or transmitted in any form or by any means, electronic, or mechanical, including photocopying, recording or by any information storage and retrieval system without permission in writing.

Contact Information: jonathanvinebooks@gmail.com

Publisher: www.ebook-pro.com

DISCLAIMER
The information presented in this book represents the views of the publisher as of the date of publication. The publisher reserves the rights to alter and update their opinions based on new conditions. This book is for informational purposes only. The author and publisher do not accept any responsibilities for any liabilities resulting from the use of this information. While every attempt has been made to verify the information provided here, the author and the publisher cannot assume any responsibility for errors, inaccuracies or omissions.

Table of contents

Introduction

The more progress we make in the food industry, the more additives and preserves we seem to use. Every single food we buy at the supermarket has at least one additive added to preserve it better, to make it look better or to taste better. But luckily over the last few years, you can see that more people have stopped eating whatever, whenever and began to become more interested in where their food comes from, how it is being produced, what it contains, and what health benefits it has. This has led to a movement that is trending more and more called *clean eating*. And that can only be a good thing, right?!

What is clean eating

This is a question I hear often, but it has such a simple answer. Clean eating is very straightforward, and it doesn't even count as a diet; it's more of a lifestyle. Clean eating is a concept that you need to embrace; a concept that revolves around the idea of knowing what your food contains and where it comes from. To put it simpler, clean eating simply means avoiding processed foods. Processing refers to food that has been processed before, such as many canned goods, white flour (and pastries made with it), and foods that have ingredients you can't identify. As a general rule, processed foods include anything from a hotdog to pasta sauce and instant oatmeal.

The problems with these foods is that they've been processed so much that part of (or all) the nutrients have been destroyed. Moreover, often additives are added to preserve the food longer, to make it look better, improve its taste, and make it irresistible. But these additives have been linked to serious health problems, including cancer, so they shouldn't be part of anyone's diet.

What to eat

Now that all the processed foods have been removed from your diet, let's see what you are allowed to eat:

Whole foods - This is simple and refers to eating fruits and vegetables fresh raw rather than including them in foods that we can live without. For instance, instead of eating banana nut muffins, eat a banana and some nuts. Also, use whole grains when cooking rather than processed ones. This includes: quinoa, bran, bulgur, and the list can go on. Focus more on grains that still have their full nutritional content and you will get more fibers and nutrients just by following this simple and handy change.

Canned foods – as long as they don't have any additives. Canned beans, tomatoes, corn or other vegetables are ok to eat as long as you read the ingredient list carefully and make sure it contains as little ingredients as possible. Buy organic cans if you can afford it as they surely have less salt and no additives.

Foods that have ingredients you can recognize easily – whenever buying something, read the label carefully and make sure you know every ingredient listed there. You will be surprised to find that many types of crackers and breads comply with clean eating rules, and this spares you a lot of time baking your own at home.

Fresh fruits and vegetables – you can indulge on these all you want. They are healthy, delicious, and can be combined into many recipes. Try to eat seasonal and buy organic or from sources that don't use additives. When out of season, you can buy frozen fruits and vegetables, but choose reliable brands and be sure to read labels.

Dried fruits

Farm range eggs

Nuts and seeds – almonds, hazelnuts, pecans, cashews, chia, pumpkin seeds, sunflower seeds – you can snack on these or use them in salads.

Healthy fats – coconut oil, avocado oil, and olive oil are what we call healthy fats, and they can be used in cooking with great success, but they can also be eaten raw, all of them having plenty of health benefits.

Dairy products – as long as they are hormone-free, come from a safe source, and are also low in fat.

Healthy sweeteners - such as honey or agave syrup – they are both allowed, but use as little as possible.

How to eat clean

Clean eating doesn't necessarily mean choosing certain foods or ingredients. It also assumes cooking at home for yourself; stop buying readymade food from supermarkets or restaurants. Cooking for yourself is cheaper and healthier because you get to control the amount of fat and seasoning you add, and you can also use quality, clean ingredients. This book includes plenty of recipes for you to try your hand at, and they are all clean, delicious and healthy, but best of all, they don't require an expert to cook them.

Another great concept of clean eating is keeping your body hydrated. This means drinking at least two liters of water daily and removing soda and carbonated drinks from your diet for good. Our body and brain is made mainly from water so we need it in order to function properly. Plus, water will help you detox your system and also conduct the nutrients better into your blood and, furthermore, to your organs and brain. This translates into better digestion, better brain functions, and an improved health.

Apart from this, think about food as a medicine and your body as a temple -treat it according to that belief. The phrase "you are what you eat" has never been truer than now! So focus on eating clean and channel your positive energy, and only then will you see a change in your lifestyle. Your health will improve, your immune system will be better, and you will feel much better overall. Your body will know how to tell you when something's wrong, but it will also know how to show you gratitude for taking care of it like you are supposed to!

How to Cook Clean

Cooking doesn't necessarily preserve the nutrients and benefits of your food. Some of these nutrients are destroyed, like vitamin C, but others are increased. So if you're not a follower of the raw trend, I suggest you cook your food wisely so it tastes great and preserves as many nutrients as possible.

Cooking clean starts with choosing clean ingredients, the ones that come from safe sources and are healthy and chemical-free. With these kinds of ingredients on hand, the job is half done already! From delicious ingredients to amazing cooked food is just one step.

Clean cooking means avoiding frying food on huge amounts of oil and focusing more on frying in small amounts of oil, steaming, stewing, and cooking on low heat. However, of all of these, steaming is the most nutritious and preserves most of the vitamins, antioxidants and fibers. Apart from the cooking technique, there's one more important thing to consider – reducing the amount of salt you use in cooking. You are free to use spices and herbs, but reduce the salt and try to enjoy food in the most natural possible way. That's when you get more flavors and nutrients that are crucial for a healthy lifestyle, healthy mind, and a healthy body.

Recipes

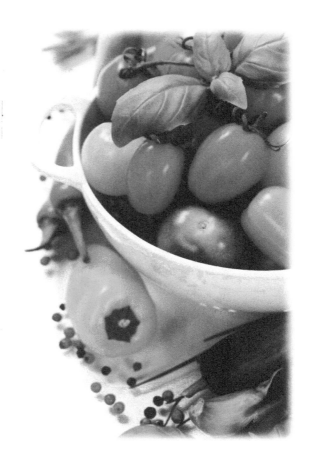

Appetizers

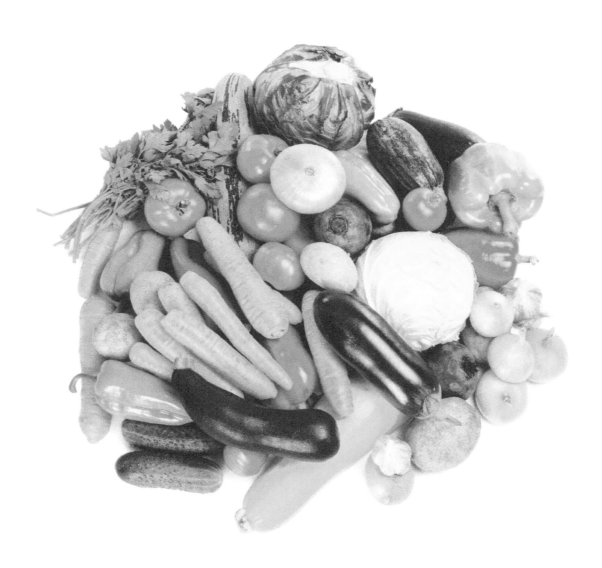

Guacamole Bruschetta

Avocado is an excellent choice of good fats and it is such a versatile fruit. In this combination it yields a rich, delicious, fresh bruschetta, perfect for a quick appetizer.

Time: 25 minutes

Servings: 8

Ingredients:

- 8 slices whole grain bread
- 1 ripe avocado
- 2 garlic cloves, minced
- 1 ripe tomato, diced
- 1 cucumber, diced
- 1 green onion, chopped
- 1 tablespoon lemon juice
- 1 tablespoon chopped cilantro
- Salt and pepper to taste

Directions:

1. Toast the bread and place them on a platter.
2. Mash the avocado into a bowl and stir in the garlic, tomato, cucumber, green onion, lemon juice and cilantro.
3. Season with salt and pepper then spoon the mixture over the bread slices.
4. Serve immediately.

Nutritional information per serving

Calories: 126

Fat: 6g

Protein: 3.9g

Carbohydrates: 16.8g

Tomato and Cheese Skewers

This is such a quick appetizer, but so pretty and fresh! The ingredient list is simple, but the result is beyond delicious. It is a dish that shines through its simplicity.

Time: 20 minutes

Servings: 6

Ingredients:

- 2 cups cherry tomatoes
- 6 oz. mozzarella, cubed
- 6 basil leaves
- Salt and pepper to taste
- 2 tablespoons olive oil
- Wooden skewers or toothpicks

Directions:

1 Place the tomatoes and mozzarella on skewers.
2 Garnish with a leaf of basil and season with salt and pepper.
3 Place the skewers on a platter and drizzle with olive oil.
4 Serve fresh.

Nutritional information per serving

Calories: 130

Fat: 9.8g

Protein: 8.6g

Carbohydrates: 3g

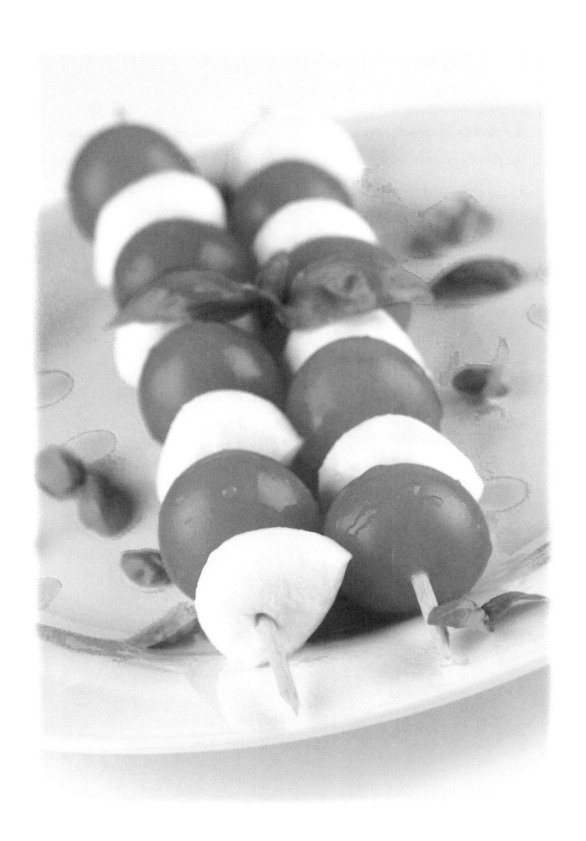

Cream Cheese Cucumber Cups

Turning cucumbers into a delicious appetizer is a great idea because they are refreshing and have a low caloric content. The filling is done with low fat cheese and parsley so it tastes great, but it is guilt free as well.

Time: 30 minutes

Servings: 4

Ingredients:

- 2 cucumbers
- ½ cup low fat cream cheese, softened
- 1 garlic clove, minced
- 1 tablespoon chopped dill
- 1 tablespoon chopped parsley
- Salt and pepper to taste

Directions:

1. Cut the cucumber into 1 1/2 –inch thick slices then scoop out part of the flesh to form cups.
2. Place them all on a platter.
3. Mix the cream cheese, garlic, dill and parsley in a bowl.
4. Add salt and pepper to taste then spoon the mixture into the cucumber cups.
5. Serve them as fresh as possible.

Nutritional information per serving

Calories: 54

Fat: 0.6g

Protein: 5.4g

Carbohydrates: 7.9g

White Bean Hummus

Easy to make and fragrant, this hummus is a crowd pleaser. Serve it with a few slices of toasted bread and tomatoes and you're up for a delicious start of the meal.

Time: 25 minutes

Servings: 6

Ingredients:

- 1 can white beans, drained
- 2 tablespoons olive oil
- 2 tablespoons water
- 2 garlic cloves
- 2 basil leaves
- ¼ cup fresh parsley
- ½ lemon, juiced
- Salt and pepper to taste
- Whole wheat bread for serving

Directions:

1. Toast the bread and place it on a platter.
2. Mix the beans, oil, water, garlic, basil, parsley and lemon juice in a blender until pureed and smooth.
3. Season with salt and pepper and pulse a few more seconds.
4. Spoon the hummus into a small bowl and place it on the platter next to the bread slices.
5. Serve immediately.

Nutritional information per serving

Calories: 165

Fat: 5g

Protein: 8g

Carbohydrates: 21g

Whole Wheat Zucchini Muffins

These savory muffins can be served as an appetizer for any meal, but they work better on a buffet. If you top them with cream cheese, they turn into a savory cupcake and can easily become the star of your meal.

Time: 40 minutes

Servings: 12

Ingredients:

- 2 cups whole wheat flour
- 1 teaspoons baking powder
- ½ teaspoon baking soda
- 1 pinch salt
- ½ cup unsweetened applesauce
- ¼ cup olive oil
- ¼ cup milk
- 1 teaspoon honey
- 2 cups grated zucchinis
- ½ cup low fat cheese, crumbled

Directions:

1 In a bowl, combine the flour, baking powder, baking soda and salt then stir in the applesauce, olive oil, milk and honey and mix well.

2 Fold in the zucchinis and cheese and spoon the mixture into 12 muffin cups lined with muffin papers.

3 Bake in the preheated oven at 350F for 20-25 minutes or until well risen and golden brown.

4 Let them cool in the pan then serve.

Nutritional information per serving

Calories: 132

Fat: 4.9g

Protein: 3.7g

Carbohydrates: 18.7g

Grilled Zucchini Rolls

Clean food diet is all about simple ingredients and amazing flavors and this recipe surely complies with that! However, you can replace the zucchinis with eggplants and create a whole new appetizer. It is a delicious recipe, regardless of the vegetable used.

Time: 35 minutes

Servings: 10

Ingredients:

- 2 zucchinis, sliced lengthwise
- 2 tablespoons olive oil
- 2 tablespoons balsamic vinegar
- Salt and pepper to taste
- 1 tablespoon chopped parsley

Directions:

1   Season the zucchini slices with salt and pepper then brush each slice with olive oil.
2   Heat a grill pan over high flame and place the zucchini slices on the grill. Cook on both sides until golden brown.
3   Transfer the zucchini in a bowl and drizzle with balsamic vinegar. Sprinkle with parsley and let them cool down.
4   Take each slice of zucchini and roll it tightly into a roll. Secure the ends with a toothpick and serve the rolls fresh.

Nutritional information per serving

Calories: 31

Fat: 2.9g

Protein: 0.5g

Carbohydrates: 1.4g

Mini Spinach Pizzas

Spinach is one of the healthiest vegetables, but hard to include in many people's diet due to its taste. However, there are ways to trick kids and even grown-ups into eating it and these pizzas do just that! They are easy to make, but delicious and versatile. After all, you can replace the spinach with other vegetable.

Time: 30 minutes

Servings: 6

Ingredients:

- 6 whole wheat pita breads
- ½ cup tomato sauce
- 1 cup spinach leaves
- 1 cup mozzarella, shredded
- Salt and pepper to taste

Directions:

1   Place the pita breads on your baking tray.
2   Brush each pita with tomato sauce and cover with spinach and mozzarella.
3   Season with salt and pepper if needed and bake in the preheated oven at 350F for 10-15 minutes or until the top is melted and crusty.
4   Serve the pizzas warm or chilled.

Nutritional information per serving

Calories: 199

Fat: 4.4g

Protein: 10.7g

Carbohydrates: 30g

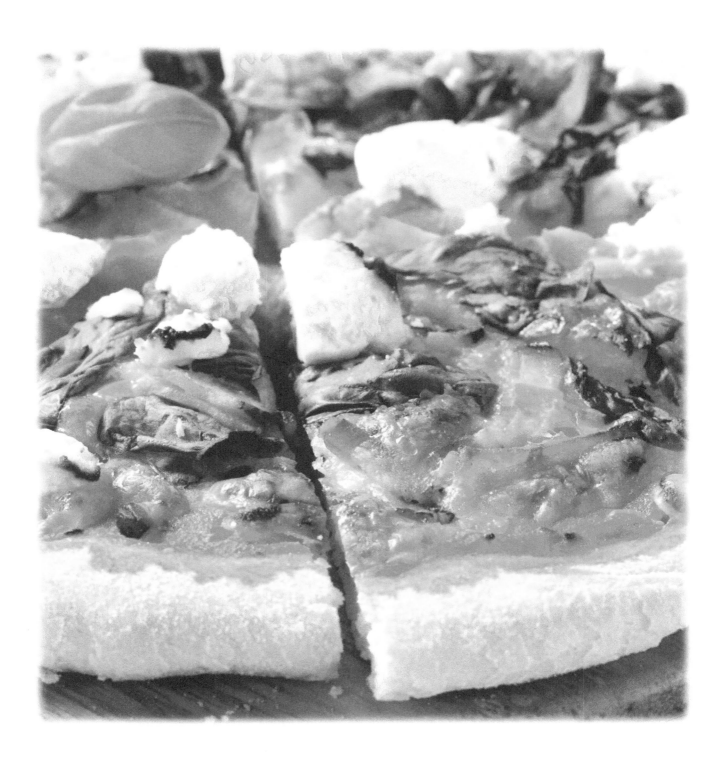

Blue Cheese Apricots

Blue cheese and fruits is a combination that never dies! The sweetness of the apricots and their delicate flavor balances the blue cheese perfectly and creates an exquisite appetizer.

Time: 25 minutes

Servings: 12

Ingredients:

- 24 dried apricots
- ½ cup low fat cream cheese
- ¼ cup blue cheese, crumbled
- 1 pinch black pepper
- Basil leaves to garnish

Directions:

1. In a bowl, mix the cream cheese and blue cheese then add a pinch of black pepper.
2. Place the apricots on a platter and drop a small dollop of cheese mixture on each apricot.
3. Garnish with a basil leaf and serve immediately.

Nutritional information per serving

Calories: 53

Fat: 1.2g

Protein: 3g

Carbohydrates: 8.4g

Wrapped Mango and Spinach Bites

It doesn't get simpler than this! This appetizer is delicious, refreshing and quick to make. But it has an exquisite feel to it and an incredible taste that comes from the contrast between the sweet and fragrant mango and salty pancetta.

Time: 25 minutes

Servings: 10

Ingredients:

- 1 ripe mango, peeled and sliced
- 2 cups spinach leaves
- Chive strands as needed
- 2 tablespoons balsamic vinegar

Directions:

1. Take 1 mango slice and a few spinach slices and wrap them together with a few chive strands.
2. Place each bundle that you make on a platter and drizzle with balsamic vinegar.
3. Serve as fresh as possible.

Nutritional information per serving

Calories: 51

Fat: 0.8g

Protein: 1.3g

Carbohydrates: 3.8g

Crusted Jalapeno Peppers

If you like spicy food, these crusted peppers will be a delicacy. They are spicy, but the heat is not overwhelming, being well balanced by the herbed cream cheese filling.

Time: 40 minutes

Servings: 10

Ingredients:

- 10 jalapeno peppers
- 1 cup low fat cream cheese
- 2 tablespoons chopped parsley
- 1 tablespoon chopped cilantro
- 1 green onion, chopped
- ¼ teaspoon garlic powder
- Salt and pepper to taste
- 2 egg whites, beaten
- ½ cup breadcrumbs

Directions:

1. Cut the top of each jalapeno pepper and remove the core and seeds.
2. In a bowl, mix the cream cheese with parsley, cilantro, green onion and garlic powder.
3. Season with salt and pepper and mix well.
4. Spoon the filling into each jalapeno pepper.
5. Dip the peppers into beaten egg whites then roll though breadcrumbs.
6. Place all the pepper in a baking tray lined with parchment paper.
7. Bake in the preheated oven at 400F for 10-15 minutes.

Nutritional information per serving

Calories: 54

Fat: 0.9g

Protein: 5g

Carbohydrates: 6.5g

Soups

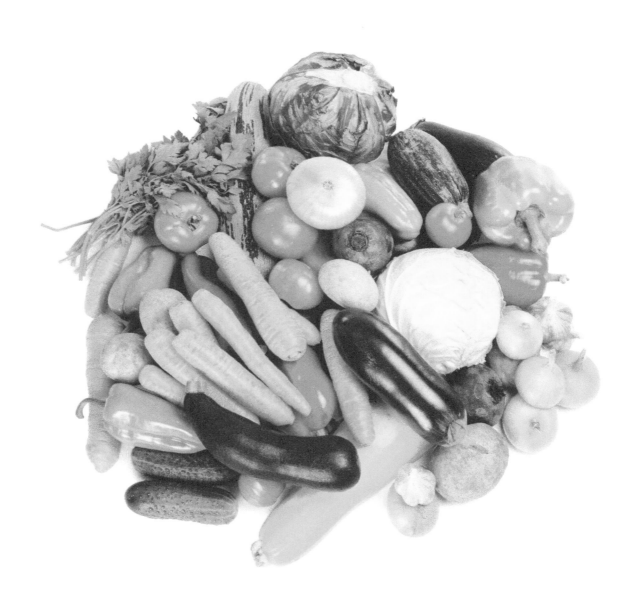

Gazpacho

This soup has Spanish origins and it is great because it uses vegetables in their natural form. No nutrient is being wasted through cooking and you get to take advantage of all of that with a bowl of soup. It's a refreshing and delicious soup, perfect for summer.

Time: 25 minutes

Servings: 6

Ingredients:

- 4 ripe tomatoes
- 2 cucumber, peeled and sliced
- 1 shallot
- 1 garlic clove
- 1 slice whole wheat bread, cubed
- 1 cup water
- 4 ice cubes
- 1 teaspoon sugar
- 1 teaspoon balsamic vinegar
- Salt and pepper to taste
- 2 tablespoons olive oil
- 2 tablespoons chopped cilantro

Directions:

1. Combine all the ingredients, except the cilantro, in a blender and pulse until smooth.
2. Season with salt and pepper then pour the soup in bowls and top with chopped cilantro.
3. Serve the soup as fresh as possible.

Nutritional information per serving

Calories: 89

Fat: 5.1g

Protein: 2.1g

Carbohydrates: 9.9g

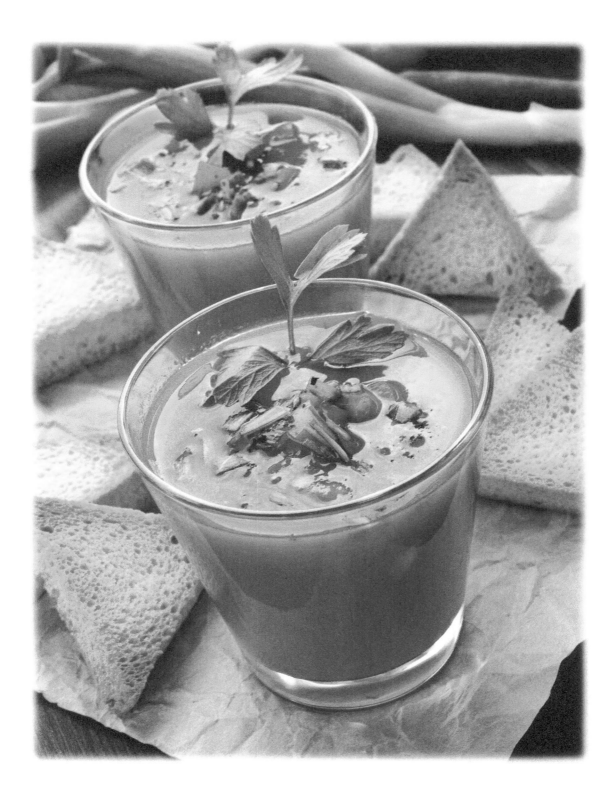

Garlicky Cauliflower Soup

Cauliflower is mild in flavor so it can take a lot of seasoning, but nothing tastes better than a touch of garlic and black pepper. It's a creamy and delicate soup and it can be made with broccoli as well.

Time: 45 minutes

Servings: 6

Ingredients:

- 2 tablespoons olive oil
- 1 onion, chopped
- 4 garlic cloves, chopped
- 1 head cauliflower, cut into florets
- 4 cups vegetable stock
- Salt and pepper to taste
- ½ lemon, juiced
- ¼ teaspoon cumin powder

Directions:

1. Heat the oil in a soup pot and stir in the onion and garlic.
2. Sauté for 2 minutes then add the cauliflower and stock.
3. Season with salt and pepper and cook the soup on medium flame for 20 minutes.
4. Add the lemon juice and cumin then puree the soup with an immersion blender.
5. Serve the soup warm.

Nutritional information per serving

Calories: 77

Fat: 4.9g

Protein: 2.3g

Carbohydrates: 7.7g

Thai Tomato Soup

This tomato soup looks common at a first glance, but once you taste it you get to feel all those Thai flavors and your taste buds go to heaven. It's a soup that doesn't need anything else, it is enough with what it has.

Time: 45 minutes

Servings: 6

Ingredients:

- 2 tablespoons olive oil
- 2 garlic cloves, chopped
- 1 shallot, chopped
- 4 heirloom tomatoes, peeled and chopped
- 1 piece 2-inch lemon grass stalk
- 1 teaspoon grated ginger
- Salt and pepper to taste
- 3 cups vegetable stock
- 1 teaspoon hot sauce

Directions:

1 Heat the oil in a soup pot and stir in the garlic and shallot.
2 Sauté for 2 minutes then add the tomatoes, lemon grass, ginger, stock and hot sauce.
3 Season with salt and pepper and cook the soup on medium flame for 20-25 minutes.
4 Remove and discard the lemongrass stalk and puree the soup with an immersion blender.
5 Serve the soup warm or chilled.

Nutritional information per serving

Calories: 78

Fat: 5g

Protein: 1g

Carbohydrates: 5.5g

White Bean and Kale Soup

The flavors of this soup are basic, but the final result is a thick, filling soup that can easily be customized to your personal taste. Replace the kale with spinach or skip it altogether. It's simple to create a new recipe using this one as a base.

Time: 1 hour
Servings: 8

Ingredients:

- 2 tablespoons olive oil
- 1 onion, chopped
- 2 garlic cloves, chopped
- 1 can white beans, drained
- 4 cups water
- 2 cups vegetable stock
- 2 tomatoes, peeled and diced
- 1 bay leaf
- ½ teaspoon cumin powder
- ½ teaspoon sweet paprika
- ½ lemon, juiced
- ¼ pound kale, shredded
- Salt and pepper to taste

Directions:

1. Heat the oil in a soup pot and stir in the onion and garlic. Sauté for 2 minutes.
2. Add the beans, water, stock and the remaining ingredients, except kale and lemon.
3. Season with salt and pepper and cook the soup for 20-30 minutes.
4. Add the kale and lemon juice and cook 10 additional minutes.

Nutritional information per serving

Calories: 146

Fat: 3.9g

Protein: 6.9g

Carbohydrates: 19.9g

Cabbage Soup

This recipe takes the basic cabbage and turns into a delicious, filling soup. The soup relies mostly on the taste of vegetables and it is light and healthy.

Time: 45 minutes

Servings: 8

Ingredients:

- 2 tablespoons olive oil
- 1 onion, chopped
- 1 red bell pepper, cored and sliced
- 1 green bell pepper, cored and sliced
- 1 head cabbage, shredded
- 3 cups water
- 2 tablespoons tomato paste
- Salt and pepper to taste
- ½ lemon, juiced
- 1 teaspoon dried thyme
- 1 tablespoon chopped cilantro

Directions:

1. Heat the oil in a soup pot and stir in the onion. Sauté for 2-3 minutes then stir in the bell peppers and cabbage.
2. Cook for 5 minutes then add the water and tomato paste and season with salt and pepper.
3. Cook the soup on medium flame for 20-30 minutes.
4. When done, stir in the lemon juice, thyme and cilantro and remove from heat.
5. Serve the soup warm.

Nutritional information per serving

Calories: 71

Fat: 3.7g

Protein: 1.7g

Carbohydrates: 9.1g

Roasted Bell Pepper Crème soup

What I love about this recipe is its creaminess and smoky flavor. It's all about grilled bell peppers in this soup and it tastes amazing.

Time: 1 ¼ hours

Servings: 8

Ingredients:

- 8 red bell peppers
- 1 tablespoon olive oil
- 1 onion, chopped
- 2 garlic cloves, chopped
- 2 tomatoes, peeled and diced
- 1 carrot, diced
- 1 parsnip, diced
- Salt and pepper to taste
- 2 cups water
- 2 cups vegetable stock
- ½ teaspoon dried thyme
- ½ teaspoon cumin powder

Directions:

1   Heat a grill pan over medium flame and place the bell peppers on the grill. Cook on all sides until browned.

2   Peel off the skin from every bell pepper and remove the core. Place aside.

3   Heat the oil in a soup pot and stir in the onion and garlic. Sauté for 2 minutes then add the bell peppers, tomatoes, carrot, parsnip, water and stock.

4   Season with salt and pepper then add the thyme and cumin powder and cook on medium flame for 30 minutes.

5   When done, puree the soup with an immersion blender and serve it warm.

Nutritional information per serving

Calories: 82

Protein: 2g

Fat: 2.3g

Carbohydrates: 14g

Cauliflower and Cashew Soup

The cashew nuts make this soup rich and thick. In terms of seasoning, the recipe keeps it simple, but that's what makes this soup so comforting and delicious – it's simple and delicate flavors.

Time: 40 minutes

Servings: 8

Ingredients:

- 1 head cauliflower, cut into florets
- 1 tablespoon olive oil
- 1 shallot, chopped
- 1 carrot, diced
- 4 cups water
- ½ cup cashew nuts, chopped
- Salt and pepper to taste
- 1 tablespoon chopped rosemary

Directions:

1. Heat the oil in a soup pot and stir in the shallot and carrot.
2. Sauté for 5 minutes then stir in the cauliflower, water and cashew nuts.
3. Cook over medium flame for 20 minutes.
4. Season with salt and pepper and puree the soup with an immersion blender.
5. Serve the soup warm, topped with rosemary.

Nutritional information per serving

Calories: 87

Fat: 5.8g

Protein: 2.1g

Carbohydrates: 5.6g

Fall Soup

This soup combines what this season has to give us best: squash, bell peppers and tomatoes. The ingredients are pureed together to create a creamy and rich soup, perfect for a comforting lunch or dinner.

Time: 45 minutes

Servings: 8

Ingredients:

- 2 tablespoons olive oil
- 1 onion, chopped
- 1 garlic clove, chopped
- 4 cups butternut squash cubes
- 1 pinch cinnamon powder
- 1 pinch ground cardamom
- ¼ teaspoon anise seeds

- 1 red bell pepper, cored and chopped
- 1 tomato, chopped
- 3 cups vegetable stock
- 1 cup water
- Salt and pepper to taste
- ¼ cup chopped walnuts to serve

Directions:

1. Heat the oil in a soup pot and stir in the onion and garlic. Sauté for 2 minutes.
2. Stir in the squash, cinnamon, cardamom, anise seeds, bell pepper and tomato then add the stock and water.
3. Season with salt and pepper and cook over medium flame for 20-30 minutes.
4. Puree the soup with an immersion blender and serve it warm, topped with walnuts.

Nutritional information per serving

Calories: 59

Fat: 3.6g

Protein: 0.7g

Carbohydrates: 3.4g

Garlic and Beet Soup

This soup has a vibrant purple color and it is a bomb of nutrients – vitamins and antioxidants, plus loads of fibers. It is a healthy soup that will help you detox your body if that is your purpose.

Time: 45 minutes

Servings: 4

Ingredients:

- 1 tablespoon olive oil
- 1 shallot, chopped
- 1 leek, sliced
- 4 garlic cloves, chopped
- 3 beets, cooked and chopped
- 2 cups vegetable stock
- 1 pinch salt
- 1 pinch cayenne pepper

Directions:

1. Heat the oil in a soup pot and stir in the shallot, leek and garlic.
2. Sauté for 5 minutes then stir in the beets and stock.
3. Season with salt and cayenne pepper and cook the soup on medium flame for 20-30 minutes.
4. Puree the soup with an immersion blender and serve it warm.

Nutritional information per serving

Calories: 86

Fat: 3.8g

Protein: 2g

Carbohydrates: 12.5g

Sweet Potato and Cauliflower Soup

The sweet potato and cauliflower are both rather sweet so they need a flavor to balance them and that flavor is a touch of lemon juice at the end. What you get is a delicious, refreshing soup, but nutritious at the same time.

Time: 50 minutes

Servings: 8

Ingredients:

- 2 tablespoons olive oil
- 1 shallot, chopped
- 1 garlic clove, chopped
- 1 head cauliflower, cut into florets
- 3 sweet potatoes, peeled and cubed
- 4 cups water
- Salt and pepper to taste
- 1 lemon, juiced
- 2 tablespoons chopped cilantro

Directions:

1 Heat the oil in a soup pot and stir in the shallot and garlic. Sauté for 2 minutes.

2 Stir in the cauliflower and sweet potatoes then add the water, salt and pepper.

3 Cook on medium flame for 30 minutes.

4 When done, stir in the lemon juice and cilantro and serve the soup warm.

Nutritional information per serving

Calories: 106

Fat: 3.6g

Protein: 1.6g

Carbohydrates: 17.8g

Salads

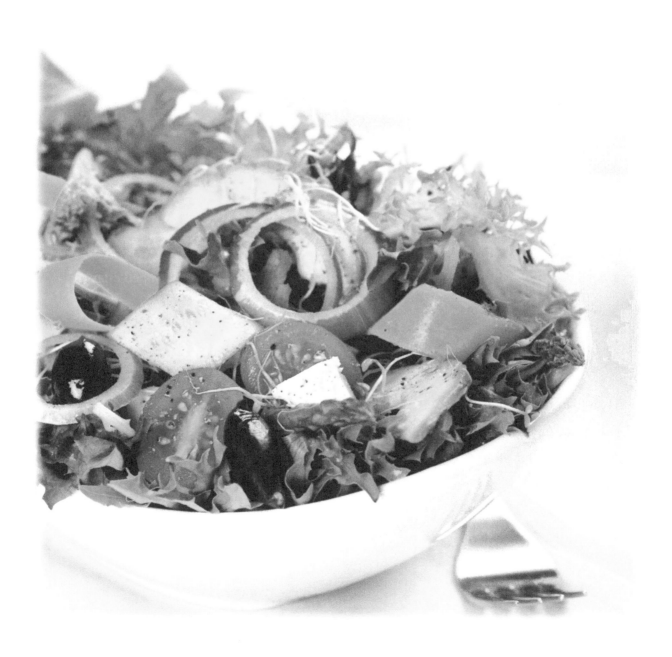

Mexican Bean Salad

Beans, corn and avocado are used to make this delicious salad. And since it's Mexican, it can't exist without a touch of spicy, can it?!

Time: 20 minutes

Servings: 6

Ingredients:

- 1 can black beans, drained
- 1 can sweet corn, drained
- 1 cucumber, sliced
- ½ cup chopped cilantro
- 1 tomato, cubed
- 1 ripe avocado, peeled and sliced
- 2 tablespoons olive oil
- 2 limes, juiced
- Salt and pepper to taste
- ½ teaspoon dried oregano

Directions:

1. Combine the beans, corn, cucumber, cilantro, tomato and avocado in a bowl.
2. Add the olive oil, lime juice and oregano then season with salt and pepper to taste.
3. Mix gently and serve the salad fresh.

Nutritional information per serving

Calories: 249

Fat: 11.8g

Protein: 8.8g

Carbohydrates: 30.4g

Light Waldorf Salad

Waldorf salad is a classic and it is one of the most nutritious salads ever, combining green leafy vegetables with fruits and vegetables and a delicious dressing.

Time: 30 minutes

Servings: 4

Ingredients:

- 1 head lettuce, shredded
- 2 red apples, sliced
- 1 celery stalk, sliced
- 2 tofu slices, grilled and cut into strips
- 2 tablespoons almond slices
- ¼ cup fat free buttermilk
- 1 teaspoon lemon zest
- 1 tablespoon lemon juice
- 1 tablespoon olive oil
- Salt and pepper to taste

Directions:

1. Combine the lettuce, apples, celery, tofu and almond slices in a salad bowl.
2. In a small glass jar, mix the buttermilk, lemon juice, olive oil plus salt and pepper to taste.
3. Drizzle this dressing over the salad and mix gently.
4. Serve the salad as fresh as possible.

Nutritional information per serving

Calories: 188

Fat: 6.1g

Protein: 17.6g

Carbohydrates: 16.1g

Balsamic Grilled Vegetable Salad

Grilling the vegetables briefly enhances their natural flavor and sweetness, but preserves the nutrients. What you get is a smoky, delicious, filling salad that can become a meal on its own or can accompany a different main dish.

Time: 35 minutes

Servings: 6

Ingredients:

- 1 zucchini, sliced
- 1 eggplant, peeled and sliced
- 2 tomatoes, sliced
- 1 red onion, sliced
- 1 carrot, finely cut lengthwise
- 2 yellow bell peppers, cored and cut in quarters

- 4 garlic cloves, chopped
- 2 tablespoons olive oil
- ¼ cup balsamic vinegar
- Salt and pepper to taste

Directions:

1. Heat a grill pan over high flame and place the vegetables on the grill, one by one.
2. Cook them until browned on each side then transfer them in a salad bowl.
3. Mix the garlic, olive oil, vinegar and salt and pepper in a bowl.
4. Drizzle the dressing over the salad and let it cool down before serving.

Nutritional information per serving

Calories: 101

Fat: 5.1g

Protein: 2.2g

Carbohydrates: 13g

Strawberry Spinach Salad

This salad will surprise you in the best possible way. It's more than a salad, it is a bomb of nutrients and a mouthful of refreshing and delicious flavors with each bite.

Time: 20 minutes

Servings: 4

Ingredients:

- 1 pound baby spinach, shredded
- 1 cup halved strawberries
- ½ cup strawberries, pureed
- ½ lemon, juiced

- 2 tablespoons olive oil
- 1 teaspoon honey
- 1 teaspoon balsamic vinegar
- Salt and pepper to taste

Directions:

1. Place the spinach on a platter. Top with halved strawberries and set aside.
2. For the dressing, mix the strawberry puree with the lemon juice, honey, balsamic vinegar and olive oil and season it with salt and pepper.
3. Drizzle the dressing over the salad and serve fresh.

Nutritional information per serving

Calories: 100

Fat: 7.5g

Protein: 3.4g

Carbohydrates: 7.6g

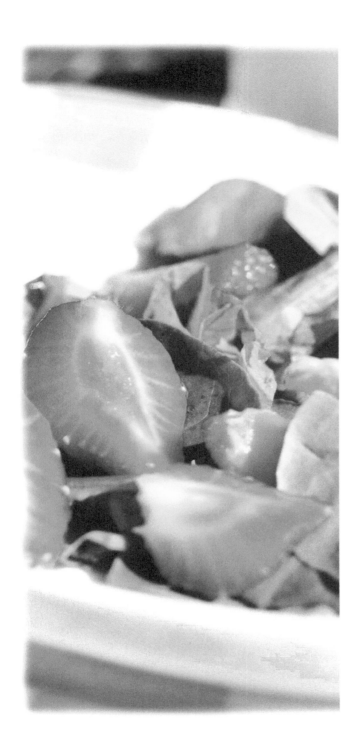

Grilled Tofu Salad

This recipe is simple and uses common ingredients, but sometimes a simple recipe like this one is all we need to feel better. The twist of this recipe is adding beans and tomatoes as well to make it more filling, but it's just as delicious.

Time: 25 minutes

Servings: 6

Ingredients:

- 3 tofu fillets
- 1 tablespoon soy sauce
- 1 teaspoon rice vinegar
- 1 head lettuce, shredded
- 2 tomatoes, sliced
- 1 cup canned black beans, drained
- 1 red onion, sliced
- ¼ cup coarsely chopped cilantro

- ½ teaspoon garlic powder
- ¼ teaspoon cumin powder
- ½ teaspoon dried oregano
- ¼ teaspoon smoked paprika
- ½ lemon, juiced
- 2 tablespoons olive oil
- ¼ cup fat free buttermilk
- Salt to taste

Directions:

1   To make the tofu, brush each slice with soy sauce and rice vinegar. Heat a grill pan over high flame and place the tofu on the hot grill. Cook on both sides until golden brown then cut into thin strips.

2   Combine the tofu, lettuce, tomatoes, black beans, red onion and cilantro in a salad bowl.

3   For the dressing, combine the buttermilk, olive oil, garlic powder, cumin powder, oregano, paprika and lemon juice in a glass jar. Cover with a lid and shake the jar well.

4   Season with salt to taste then drizzle the dressing over the salad.

5   Serve the salad fresh.

Nutritional information per serving

Calories: 180

Protein:8.4g

Fat: 5.3g

Carbohydrates: 26.2g

Multi Veggie Chickpea Salad

This salad is so filling that it could easily become a meal on its own. The chickpeas are the base of the recipes and the only compulsory ingredient. The rest can be replaced or skipped to create a salad that best fits your taste.

Time: 20 minutes

Servings: 6

Ingredients:

- 1 can chickpeas, drained
- 1 red bell pepper, cored and sliced
- 1 green bell pepper, cored and sliced
- 1 tomato, sliced
- 1 avocado, peeled and sliced
- 1 cup shredded cabbage
- ½ cup chopped cilantro
- Salt and pepper to taste
- ½ lemon, juiced
- 1 tablespoon balsamic vinegar
- 1 tablespoon olive oil

Directions:

1. In a bowl, mix the chickpeas, bell peppers, tomato, avocado, cabbage and cilantro in a salad bowl.
2. Add salt and pepper to taste then stir in the lemon juice, vinegar and olive oil.
3. Serve the salad fresh.

<u>Nutritional information per serving</u>

Calories: 228

Fat: 11g

Protein: 7.7g

Carbohydrates: 26.6g

Spinach and Avocado Salad with Poppy Seed Dressing

The great thing about this recipe is the contrast between the creamy avocado and crunchy poppy seeds. It is this contrast that creates the flavor profile of the salad, the lemon juice only enhancing it.

Time: 20 minutes

Servings: 6

Ingredients:

- 1 pound baby spinach
- 1 avocado, peeled and sliced
- 2 tablespoons sliced almonds
- ½ lemon, juiced
- 1 teaspoon lemon zest

- 1 tablespoon poppy seed
- 1 teaspoon honey
- 1 teaspoon apple cider vinegar
- 1 tablespoon olive oil
- Salt and pepper to taste

Directions:

1 Combine the spinach, avocado and sliced almonds on a platter.
2 In a bowl, mix the lemon juice, lemon zest, poppy seeds, honey, vinegar, olive oil, salt and pepper in a glass jar. Cover with a lid and shake the jar well.
3 Drizzle the dressing over the salad and serve it as fresh as possible.

Nutritional information per serving

Calories: 129

Fat: 10.8g

Protein: 3.5g

Carbohydrates: 7.4g

Radish and Cucumber Creamy Salad

The dressing of this salad is creamy and rich, although low in fat. Combined with cucumbers and radishes it create a refreshing salad that works great as a side dish for a steak, although I would serve it even as a stand-alone meal during summer.

Time: 15 minutes

Servings: 4

Ingredients:

- 2 cucumbers, sliced
- 15 radishes, sliced
- ¼ cup low fat yogurt
- 1 garlic, minced
- 1 tablespoon olive oil
- Salt and pepper to taste

Directions:

1. Mix the yogurt, garlic, olive oil, salt and pepper in a bowl.
2. Add the cucumbers and radishes and mix gently.
3. Serve the salad fresh.

Nutritional information per serving

Calories: 67

Fat: 3.9g

Protein: 2g

Carbohydrates: 7.4g

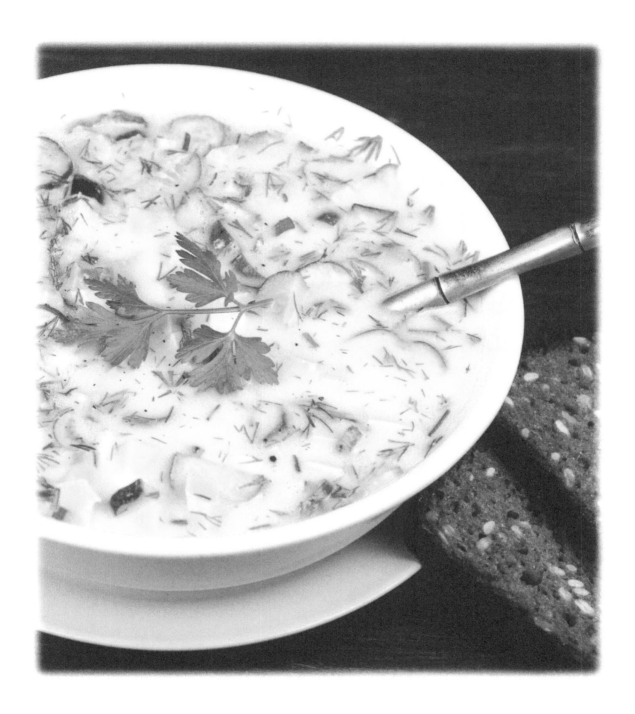

Tabbouleh Quinoa Salad

Tabbouleh is a well-known salad that combines vegetables with herbs, but this recipe adds a twist to the classic – uses quinoa instead of bulgur. They are both healthy grains, but quinoa has more fibers and nutrients overall and therefore it is the better choice.

Time: 35 minutes

Servings: 6

Ingredients:

- 1 cup quinoa, rinsed
- 1 cup vegetable stock
- 1 cup water
- 1 red onion, sliced
- 2 tomatoes, diced
- 4 mint leaves, chopped
- 2 green onions, chopped
- 1 cup chopped Parsley
- ½ cup chopped cilantro
- 4 basil leaves, chopped
- 2 tablespoons olive oil
- 1 teaspoon cumin seeds
- 1 lemon, juiced
- Salt and pepper to taste

Directions:

1. Combine the quinoa, stock and water in a saucepan and bring to a boil over medium flame.
2. Cook until most of the liquid has been absorbed.
3. Transfer the quinoa into a salad bowl and add the red onion, tomatoes, mint, green onions, parsley, cilantro and basil leaves.
4. Stir in the olive oil, cumin seeds and lemon juice then season with salt and pepper.
5. Serve the salad fresh.

Nutritional information per serving

Calories: 165

Protein: 5.1g

Fat: 6.6g

Carbohydrates: 22.4g

Pear and Arugula Salad

Although it sounds like a weird combination at first, this salad is delicious. It combines the pears with arugula and walnuts and the final result is rich and filling.

Time: 20 minutes

Servings: 4

Ingredients:

- 1 pound arugula
- 2 pears, sliced
- ½ lemon, juiced
- 1 teaspoon honey
- 1 teaspoon apple cider vinegar
- 1 tablespoon Dijon mustard
- Salt and pepper to taste
- ¼ cup walnuts, chopped

Directions:

1 Place the arugula on a platter. Arrange the pear slices over the arugula.

2 In a small glass jar, mix the lemon juice, honey, vinegar and mustard. Add salt and pepper to taste and cover the jar with a lid.

3 Shake well then drizzle the dressing over the salad.

4 Top with walnuts and serve immediately.

Nutritional information per serving

Calories: 145

Fat: 5.7g

Protein: 5.4g

Carbohydrates: 22.8g

Main Dishes

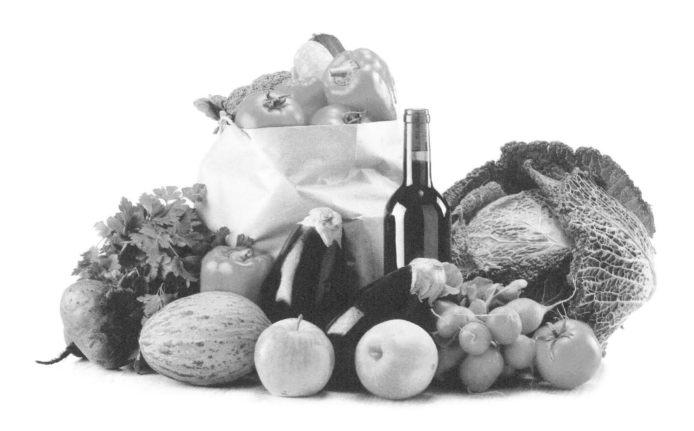

Buttermilk Marinated Tofu Kebabs

Turn on that grill and make these delicious kebabs. The buttermilk flavors the tofu and makes it tender and melt-in-your-mouth. Feel free to add any seasoning you want to the buttermilk for even more aroma.

Time: 1 ½ hours

Servings: 6

Ingredients:

- 3 slices tofu, cubed
- 1 cup fat free buttermilk
- 1 tablespoon olive oil
- 1 teaspoon Worcestershire sauce
- 1 tablespoon chopped rosemary
- ½ teaspoon smoked paprika
- Salt and pepper to taste

Directions:

1 Combine the tofu, buttermilk, olive oil, Worcestershire sauce, rosemary and paprika in a bowl.
2 Add salt and pepper to taste and place the bowl in the fridge for 1 hour.
3 After one hour, remove the bowl from the fridge and place the tofu cubes on skewers.
4 Heat your electric grill to high and place the skewers on the grill.
5 Cook on all sides for 2-3 minutes or until browned.
6 Serve the kebabs warm.

Nutritional information per serving

Calories: 82

Fat: 5.1g

Protein:5.2g

Carbohydrates:1.7g

Ginger Glazed Tofu

Tofu is as versatile as meat, but it has a higher nutritional profile. It also has a mild taste and can take a lot of seasoning. This recipe does just that – seasons tofu perfectly to create an Asian flavored dish that can be served as lunch, dinner or even used to make sandwiches.

Time: 35 minutes

Servings: 4

Ingredients:

- 4 firm tofu slices
- 2 tablespoons raw honey
- 2 tablespoons grated ginger
- 2 garlic cloves, minced
- 1 tablespoon Dijon mustard
- 1 tablespoon soy sauce

Directions:

1 In a small bowl, mix the honey, ginger, garlic, mustard and soy sauce.
2 Brush tofu slices with this mixture and place them on a baking tray lined with parchment paper.
3 Bake in the preheated oven at 350F for 20-25 minutes until golden brown.
4 Serve the tofu warm with your favorite side dish.

Nutritional information per serving

Calories:175

Fat:6.6g

Protein:13.5g

Carbohydrates:14.7g

Asian Tofu Lettuce Wraps

Tofu is a great meat replacer for vegetarians because it has a high amount of proteins. Plus, its texture and cooking style is similar to chicken or turkey so tofu eases the transition from meat to vegetarian while offering you more nutrients than meat does.

Time: 25 minutes

Servings: 6

Ingredients:

- 1 tablespoon olive oil
- 1 pound firm tofu, crumbled
- 2 garlic cloves, minced
- 1 shallot, chopped
- 1 tablespoon soy sauce
- 1 teaspoon hoisin sauce
- Lettuce leaves for serving

- 1 tablespoon rice vinegar
- ½ teaspoon Sriracha sauce
- 2 green onions, chopped
- ¼ cup peanuts, chopped
- Salt and pepper to taste

Directions:

1 Heat the oil in a skillet and add the crumbled tofu.

2 Season with a pinch of salt and pepper and cook the tofu, stirring often, until most of the juices evaporate.

3 Add the garlic, shallot, soy sauce, hoisin sauce, vinegar and Sriracha and continue cooking 5-10 additional minutes.

4 When done, stir in the green onions and peanuts then spoon the mixture into lettuce leaves and serve.

Nutritional information per serving

Calories: 116   Protein:8.1g

Fat:8.5g

Carbohydrates:3.6g

Mediterranean Stuffed Eggplants

Quick and easy to make, this dish is a summer masterpiece. It combines what summer has to offer best: tomatoes, eggplants and fresh cheese in order to create a filling, juicy, delicious dish that tastes amazing warm, but even better chilled.

Time: 45 minutes

Servings: 4

Ingredients:

- 2 eggplants
- 2 tablespoons olive oil
- 1 shallot
- 2 garlic cloves, chopped
- 2 roasted red bell peppers, chopped

- 1 tomato, diced
- ¼ cup chopped parsley
- 1 teaspoon dried basil
- Salt and pepper to taste
- 6 oz. low fat mozzarella cheese

Directions:

1. Cut the eggplants in half lengthwise and scoop out the flesh, leaving the skins intact.
2. Chop the flesh into small pieces.
3. Heat the oil in a skillet and stir in the shallot and garlic. Sauté for 2 minutes then add the chopped eggplants.
4. Cook 5 additional minutes then remove from heat and stir in the bell peppers, tomato, parsley and basil.
5. Season with salt and pepper then spoon the mixture into the eggplant skins.
6. Top with mozzarella cheese and place the eggplant halves in a baking tray lined with parchment paper.
7. Bake in the preheated oven at 350F for 20-30 minutes.

Nutritional information per serving

Calories: 192

Fat: 11.1g

Protein: 7.5g

Carbohydrates: 19.4g

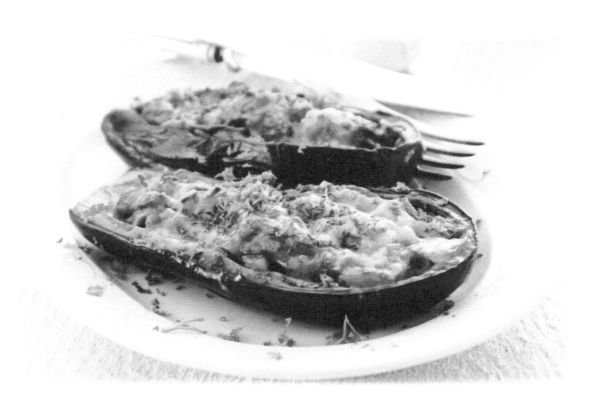

Herbed Quinoa Cakes

These patties are moist and delicious and can be served simple, with a garlic sauce or used in sandwiches for a takeaway lunch.

Time: 50 minutes

Servings: 14

Ingredients:

- 2 cups cooked quinoa
- 4 eggs, beaten
- 1 shallot, chopped
- 2 garlic cloves, chopped
- 1 cup whole wheat breadcrumbs
- Salt and pepper to taste
- 1 carrot, grated
- 2 tablespoons oil for frying

Directions:

1. Combine the quinoa, eggs, shallot, garlic, breadcrumbs and carrot in a bowl.
2. Season with salt and pepper then mix well.
3. Heat the oil in a large skillet then form small patties and place them in the hot pan.
4. Fry on both sides until golden brown.
5. Serve the patties warm.

Nutritional information per serving

Calories: 142

Fat: 4.7g

Protein: 5.8g

Carbohydrates: 19.5g

Lemon Crusted Tofu

The lemon crust is crisp and fragrant, just what this mild tofu needs to get a nice kick. Serve the dish simple or with a salad on one side and your taste buds will be grateful for such a refreshing taste.

Time: 35 minutes

Servings: 4

Ingredients:

- 4 tofu slices
- 1 lemon, juiced
- ½ cup breadcrumbs
- 2 tablespoons chopped parsley
- 1 teaspoon lemon zest
- Salt and pepper to taste
- 1 tomato, diced

Directions:

1. In a bowl, combine the lemon juice, breadcrumbs, parsley, lemon zest and tomato.
2. Place the tofu in a baking tray lined with parchment paper.
3. Top each tofu slice with the breadcrumb mixture and bake in the preheated oven at 350F for 20 minutes.
4. Serve the tofu warm with your favorite side dish, although I recommend a simple salad.

Nutritional information per serving

Calories: 188

Fat: 7.1g

Protein:14.9g

Carbohydrates:15.1g

Meatless Chili

Chili is usually made with beef or pork, but this recipe skips the meat and creates a filling, flavorful dish without any kind of animal protein. It's a sweet, spicy, flavorful dish, great for the entire family.

Time: 1 hour
Servings: 8

Ingredients:

- 2 tablespoons olive oil
- 1 onion, chopped
- 2 garlic cloves, chopped
- 2 red bell peppers, cored and diced
- 1 carrot, diced
- 1 can black beans, drained
- 1 can cannellini beans, drained
- 1 can diced tomatoes
- 1 cup vegetable stock
- 1 teaspoon cumin powder
- ½ teaspoon dried oregano
- ¼ teaspoon smoked paprika
- 2 bay leaves
- Salt and pepper to taste
- Chopped cilantro for serving

Directions:

1   Heat the oil in a large heavy pot and stir in the onion and garlic. Sauté for 2 minutes.

2   Stir in the bell peppers and carrot and sauté 2 additional minutes.

3   Stir in the beans, tomatoes, stock, cumin, oregano, paprika and bay leaves then add salt and pepper to taste.

4   Cook the chili on low heat for 40 minutes.

5   Serve the chili warm, topped with chopped cilantro.

Nutritional information per serving

Calories: 213

Fat:4.3g

Protein:11.4g

Carbohydrates:33.7g

Zucchini Oven Fries

Once you taste this recipe you will get hooked! These fries taste amazing warm, but they are even better chilled. It is a simple summer, but like all recipes of this kind, it truly shines!

Time: 40 minutes

Servings: 6

Ingredients:

Zucchini fries:

- 2 zucchinis, sliced

- 1 cup fat free buttermilk

- 1 tablespoon chopped dill

- Salt and pepper to taste

- 1 cup whole wheat breadcrumbs

- 2 tablespoons grated Parmesan

Garlic sauce:

- ½ cup low fat yogurt

- 4 garlic cloves, minced

- 1 cucumber, grated

- 1 pinch salt

Directions:

1 To make the zucchini fries, in a bowl, combine the buttermilk, dill, salt and pepper then add the zucchini slices.

2 Toss around to evenly coat them in the buttermilk mixture.

3 Mix the breadcrumbs with the Parmesan. Take each zucchini slice and roll it through breadcrumbs then place them all on a baking tray lined with parchment paper.

4 Bake in the preheated oven at 400F for 10 minutes.

5 For the sauce, mix all the ingredients in a bowl.

6 Serve the fries dipped into the garlic sauce.

Nutritional information per serving

Calories: 129

Fat: 2.8g

Protein: 9g

Carbohydrates: 18.2g

Greek Vegetarian Burgers

Burgers don't have to be fatty and greasy like the ones you buy in a fast food in order to be tasty. This recipe uses lentils and beans to create a moist, flavorful and filling vegetarian burger that has Greek flavors – basil, oregano and feta cheese for its saltiness.

Time: 45 minutes
Servings: 8

Ingredients:

- 2 cups cooked lentils
- 1 cup canned beans, drained
- 1 tablespoon olive oil
- 1 onion, finely chopped
- 1 carrot, grated
- ½ cup whole wheat breadcrumbs
- 1 teaspoon dried thyme
- 1 teaspoon dried basil
- ½ teaspoon dried oregano
- ½ teaspoon garlic powder
- 2 eggs
- Salt and pepper to taste
- 1 cup feta cheese, crumbled
- Whole wheat burger buns

Directions:

1 Place the beans in a food processor and pulse until smooth.

2 Transfer the beans in a bowl and stir in the rest of the ingredients.

3 Adjust the taste with salt and pepper then wet your hands and form small burgers.

4 Place them on a baking tray lined with parchment paper and bake in the preheated oven at 400F for 10-15 minutes just until they begin to turn golden brown.

5 Serve the burgers warm with your favorite toppings.

Nutritional information per serving

Calories: 282

Fat: 7.5g

Protein: 17.6g

Carbohydrates: 36.5g

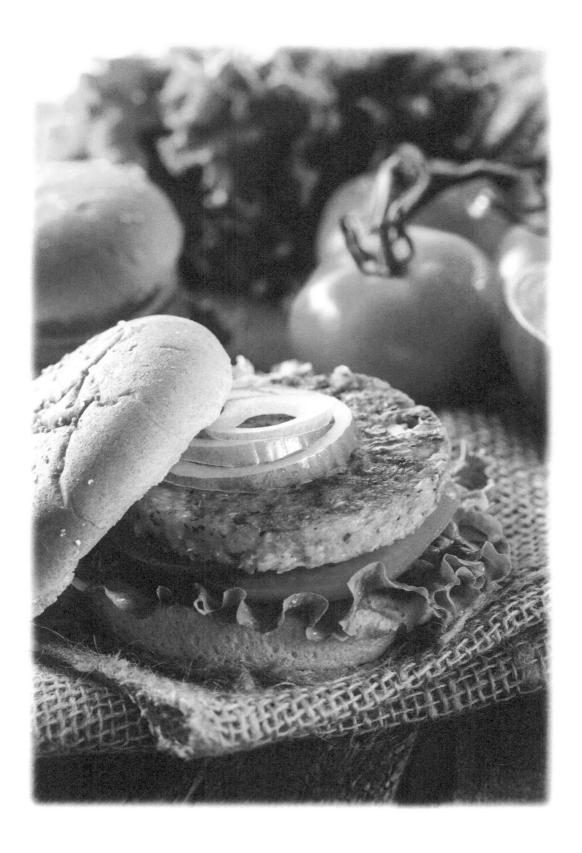

Quinoa Stuffed Bell Peppers

When it comes to versatile recipes, nothing beats this one. I've made these stuffed peppers with whole wheat, with quinoa, with bulgur and the list can go. And they turned out amazing every single time!

Time: 1 ¼ hours
Servings: 6

Ingredients:

- 6 red bell peppers
- 1 cup quinoa
- 2 cups vegetable stock
- 1 carrot, grated
- 1 shallot, chopped

- 1 tomato, diced
- 2 tablespoons chopped parsley
- Salt and pepper to taste
- ½ cup low fat mozzarella, shredded

Directions:

1 Cut the top of each bell pepper and remove the core.
2 Place the peppers in a baking tray and place aside.
3 Combine the quinoa and stock in a saucepan and cook over low heat until all the liquid has been absorbed.
4 Remove from heat and stir in the carrot, shallot, tomato and parsley.
5 Season with salt and pepper then spoon the mixture into each bell pepper.
6 Top with mozzarella and place the tray in the preheated oven at 330F foe 40-50 minutes or until the peppers are tender.
7 Serve the peppers warm.

Nutritional information per serving

Calories: 170

Fat: 3.7g

Protein: 8g

Carbohydrates: 26.4g

Desserts

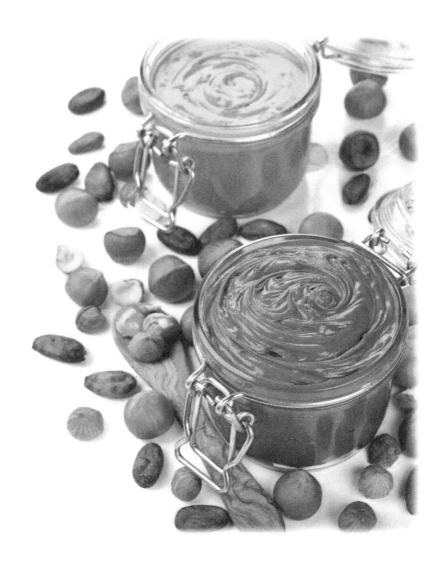

Two-Ingredient Oatmeal Cookies

You will be surprised to discover some amazing cookies, despite their short ingredient list. Only bananas and rolled oats are used, but the final result is nutritious, healthy and delicious. The recipe itself can be customized by adding chocolate chips or some dried fruits.

Time: 35 minutes

Servings: 2 dozen

Ingredients:

- 2 ripe bananas, mashed
- 2 cups rolled oats

Directions:

1. Mix the bananas and rolled oats in a bowl.
2. Drop spoonfuls of this mixture on a baking tray lined with parchment paper and bake in the preheated oven at 350F for 15-20 minutes.
3. Let them cool in the pan before serving.

Nutritional information per serving

Calories: 42

Fat: 0.5g

Protein: 1.2g

Carbohydrates: 8.2g

Clean Chocolate Soufflé

Yes, you read that right! Chocolate soufflé can be part of your diet if you prepare it following this recipe. It yields a delicious, airy soufflé with an intense taste. Just top it with some fresh fruits and your dessert is done!

Time: 40 minutes

Servings: 4

Ingredients:

- ¼ cup natural cocoa powder
- 2 tablespoons whole wheat flour
- ½ cup low fat milk
- ½ cup honey
- 4 egg whites
- 1 teaspoon lemon juice

Directions:

1. In a bowl, mix the egg whites with the lemon juice until fluffy then add the honey and keep mixing until glossy and stiff.
2. Fold in the cocoa powder, flour and milk then pour the mixture into 4 individual ramekins.
3. Bake in the preheated oven at 350F for 15-20 minutes until well risen.
4. Serve the soufflés warm.

Nutritional information per serving

Calories: 172

Fat: 0.4g

Protein: 5.2g

Carbohydrates: 39g

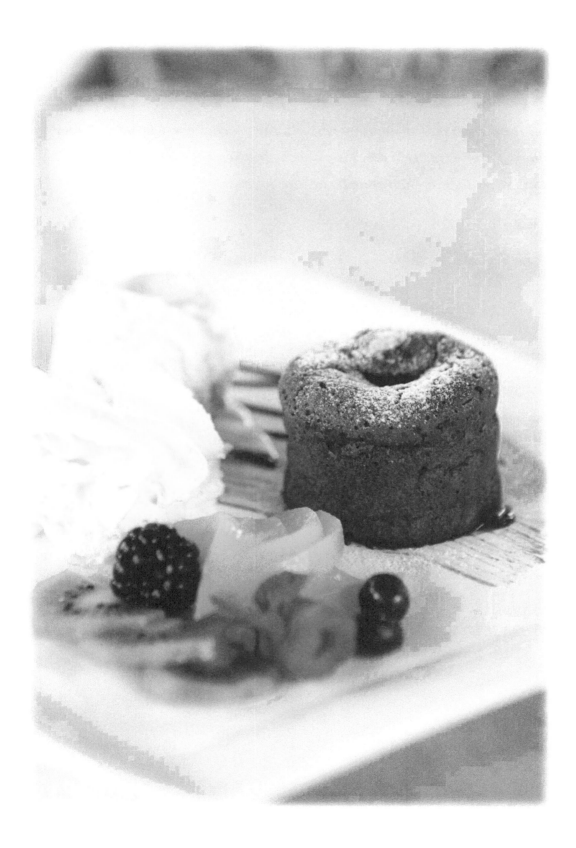

Grilled Peaches

Grilling these peaches turns them into an amazing dessert! The peaches are delicate and juicy and combined with the smoky flavor of the grill they taste even better. Serve them drizzles with honey and topped with almond slices for more flavor and a texture contrast.

Time: 25 minutes

Servings: 2

Ingredients:

- 4 peaches, halved
- ½ teaspoon cinnamon powder
- 2 tablespoons raw honey
- 2 tablespoons almond slices

Directions:

1. Sprinkle the peaches with cinnamon powder.
2. Heat your grill pan over medium flame and place the peaches on the grill.
3. Cook the peaches on both sides until browned then transfer them on a serving platter and drizzle with honey.
4. Top with almond slices and serve immediately.

Nutritional information per serving

Calories: 320

Fat: 15.5g

Protein: 7.8g

Carbohydrates: 42g

Fruit Kebabs

These colorful and fresh fruit kebabs are a summer delicacy! You can sue any fruit you want, but choose different colors to create a contrast.

Time: 35 minutes

Servings: 6

Ingredients:

- 1 cup red grapes
- 1 cantaloupe, cubed
- 2 cups fresh strawberries
- Mint leaves as needed
- ½ lemon, juiced

Directions:

1. Place the red grapes, cantaloupe and strawberries on wooden skewers.
2. Garnish each kebab with mint leaves then drizzle them with lemon juice.
3. Serve the kebabs fresh.

Nutritional information per serving

Calories: 32

Fat: 0.2g

Protein: 0.6g

Carbohydrates: 7.8g

Chocolate Covered Strawberries

Although a classic, this recipe never stops to impress with its amazing taste! Plus, it looks amazing and it matches any type of meal because it is a well-balanced combination between a rich chocolate and a refreshing fruit.

Time: 25 minutes

Servings: 4

Ingredients:

- 1 pound fresh strawberries
- 1 cup dark chocolate chips

Directions:

1. Melt the chocolate over a hot water bath.
2. Dip each strawberry into the melted chocolate and place them on a baking tray lined with parchment paper.
3. Refrigerate 10 minutes to allow the chocolate to set.
4. Serve immediately.

Nutritional information per serving

Calories: 176

Fat: 8.3g

Protein: 2.8g

Carbohydrates: 28.7g

Chocolate Popsicles

All you want during summer is something to cool you off and these popsicles are just the right thing! They are rich and delicious, but skinny and as healthy as a dessert can get.

Time: 4 hours

Servings: 6

Ingredients:

- 6 tablespoons natural cocoa powder
- 1 avocado
- 1 ½ cups low fat coconut milk
- ½ cup honey
- 1 teaspoon lemon juice
- 1 teaspoon vanilla extract

Directions:

1. Combine all the ingredients in a blender and pulse until smooth.
2. Pour the mixture into 6 popsicle molds and freeze them at least 3 hours.
3. To remove them from their molds, sink them in hot water for a few seconds.
4. Serve immediately.

Nutritional information per serving

Calories: 209

Fat: 10g

Protein: 1.7g

Carbohydrates: 32.3g

Skinny Homemade Nutella

We all love Nutella, don't we?! But the store bought one is not as healthy as we'd like so here is a version that is homemade and has less calories and more nutrients without losing the well-known Nutella taste.

Time: 20 minutes

Servings: 6

Ingredients:

- 1 cup hazelnuts
- ¾ cup dark chocolate chips
- ¾ cup light coconut milk
- 3 tablespoons raw honey
- 1 pinch salt

Directions:

1 Combine the hazelnuts, chocolate chips, honey and salt in a blender.

2 Pulse until ground then gradually stir in the coconut milk, mixing well for a few minutes until smooth.

3 Spoon the Nutella into a glass jar and store it in the fridge for 3-4 days.

4 Serve it simple or with fruit and even light crackers.

Nutritional information per serving

Calories: 249

Fat: 18.7g

Protein: 3.6g

Carbohydrates: 22.4g

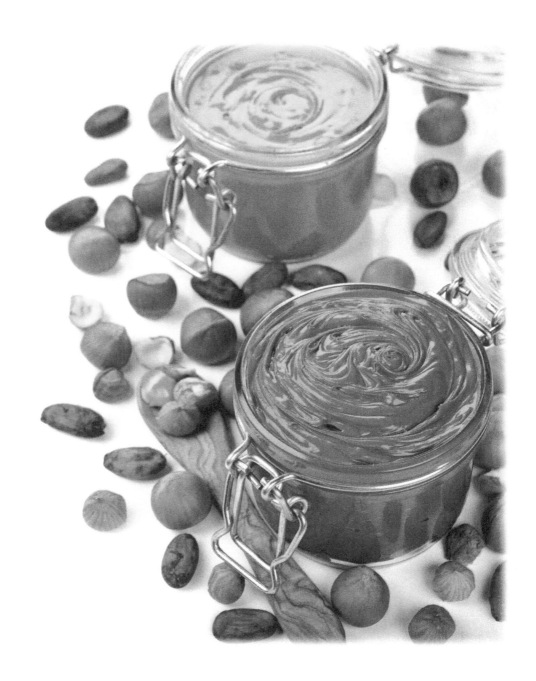

Dried Fruit Granola

Granola is amazing because it can be served as breakfast, but it also makes an excellent quick dessert if you pair it with yogurt or milk. This recipe uses dried fruits and rolled oats, but it has less fats and sweeteners so it is healthier.

Time: 45 minutes

Servings: 20

Ingredients:

- 4 cups rolled oats
- 1 cup almond slices
- 1 cup coconut flakes
- ½ cup dried raisins
- ¼ cup dried cranberries
- ¼ cup dried pineapple cubes
- 1 pinch cinnamon powder
- ¼ cup raw honey
- ¼ cup coconut oil

Directions:

1 In a bowl, combine the oats, coconut flakes, almond slices, raisins, cranberries, pineapple and cinnamon and mix well.
2 In a saucepan, mix the honey and coconut oil and melt them together.
3 Drizzle this mixture over the oats and mix well then spread the mixture on a baking tray lined with parchment paper.
4 Bake in the preheated oven at 350F for 30-35 minutes.
5 When done, remove from the oven and store in an airtight container or jar for up to 2 weeks.

Nutritional information per serving

Calories: 174

Fat: 7.7g

Protein: 3.5g

Carbohydrates: 19.3g

Banana Strawberry Smoothie

With such an amazing taste, this smoothie qualifies as dessert! It's thick and rich, fragrant and delicious, but also healthy and nutritious. If you ask me, this is the perfect dessert for a healthy lifestyle.

Time: 10 minutes
Servings: 4

Ingredients:

- 2 ripe bananas
- ½ cup fresh or frozen strawberries
- 2 tablespoons wheat germ
- 1 cup almond milk
- ½ cup low fat yogurt
- 1 tablespoon raw honey

Directions:

1. Combine all the ingredients in a blender and pulse until smooth.
2. Pour the mixture into serving glasses and serve it as fresh as possible as it tends to change color in time and lose nutrients.

Nutritional information per serving

Calories: 232

Fat: 14.7g

Protein: 3g

Carbohydrates: 26.1g

Caramelized Pineapple

Pineapple is one of the healthiest tropical fruits you can easily find at the supermarket. It has plenty of antioxidants and vitamins to help your immune system toughen up and it tastes amazing. But this recipe combines it with honey and grills it until caramelized. What a delicacy!

Time: 20 minutes

Servings: 4

Ingredients:

- 4 pineapple slices
- 4 tablespoons raw honey
- 4 mint leaves, chopped
- 2 tablespoons lemon juice
- Frozen yogurt for serving

Directions:

1 Mix the honey, mint and lemon juice in a bowl.

2 Brush the pineapple slices with this mixture.

3 Heat a grill pan over high flame and place the pineapple on the grill.

4 Cook on both sides until browned then transfer on serving plates and top with a scoop of frozen yogurt.

5 Serve immediately.

Nutritional information per serving

Calories: 189

Fat: 0.3g

Protein: 1.4g

Carbohydrates: 40g

Conclusion

Clean eating is a challenge given the amount of processed foods you can find on the market, but there are still gems to be found out there and you can still do it yourself. It sounds harder than it actually is and once you get started and taste a real clean food and get to testify its benefits later on, there's nothing stopping you. Clean eating improves your health, it boosts your immune system, it helps you think better, it makes your skin look better, it makes your hair shine and your tummy feel much better as well. And all with a few simple lifestyle changes! Not in a month or two, but now! Now is the time for that change, now is the time to feel better, do this for yourself and be grateful for it!

More books in *Special Vegetarian Diet* series:

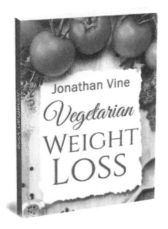 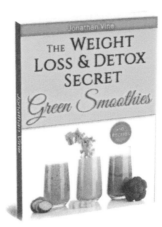 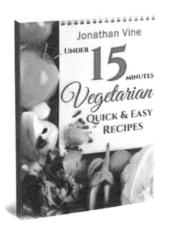

CPSIA information can be obtained at www.ICGtesting.com
Printed in the USA
BVOW10*1817190815

414006BV00013B/31/P